THIS
SEX CALEND
BELONGS TO:

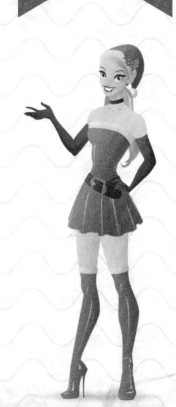

....

AND

....

NO EXCHANGE - NO REFUNDS
18+ ADULTS ONLY 18+

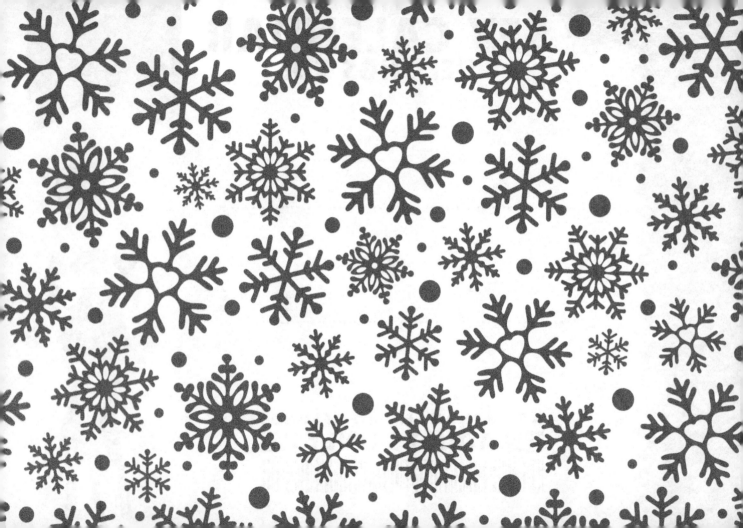

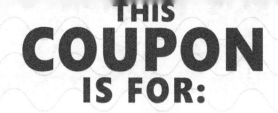

THIS COUPON IS FOR:

MASSAGE MY...

MASSAGE WHATEVER I WANT YOU TO FOR 15 MINUTES

1

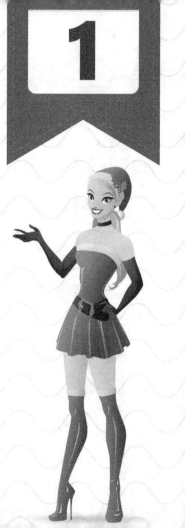

NO EXCHANGE - NO REFUNDS

18+ ADULTS ONLY 18+

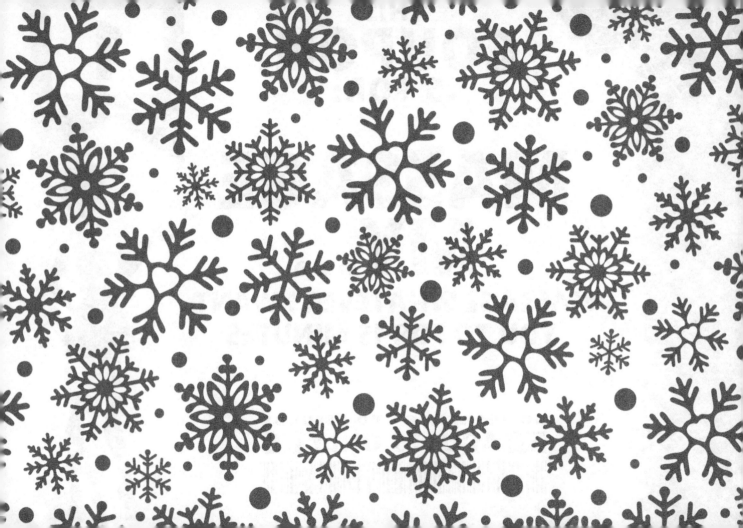

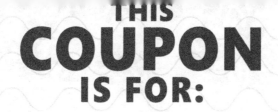

THIS COUPON IS FOR:

2

SURPRISE ORAL SEX

YOUR PARTNER COMMITS TO SURPRISING YOU WITH ORAL SEX WITHIN THE NEXT 24 HOURS

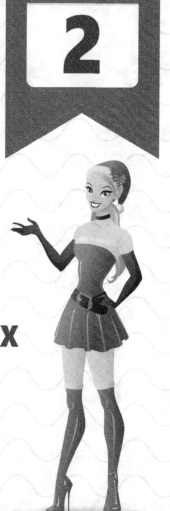

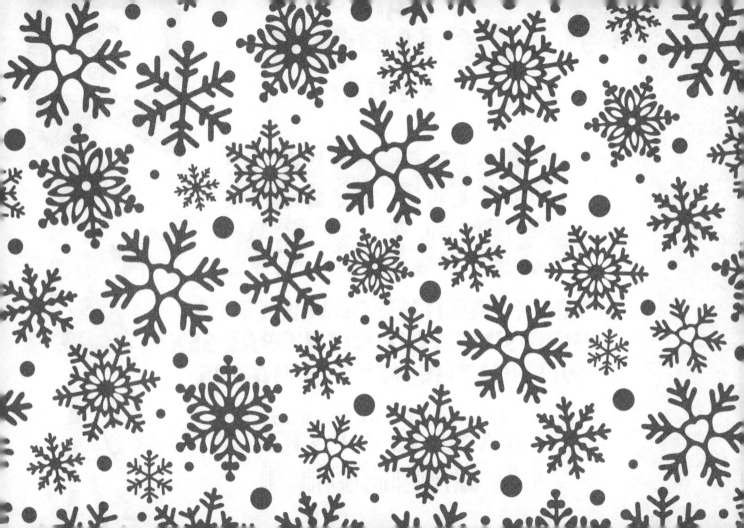

THIS COUPON IS FOR:

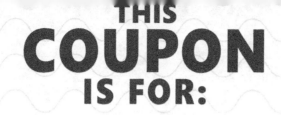

3

SEE AND DO

YOUR PARTNER CHOOSES A PORNO MOVIE AND YOU BOTH TRY TO REENACT IT FOR 10 MINUTES

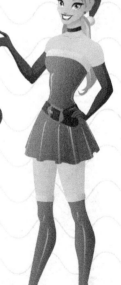

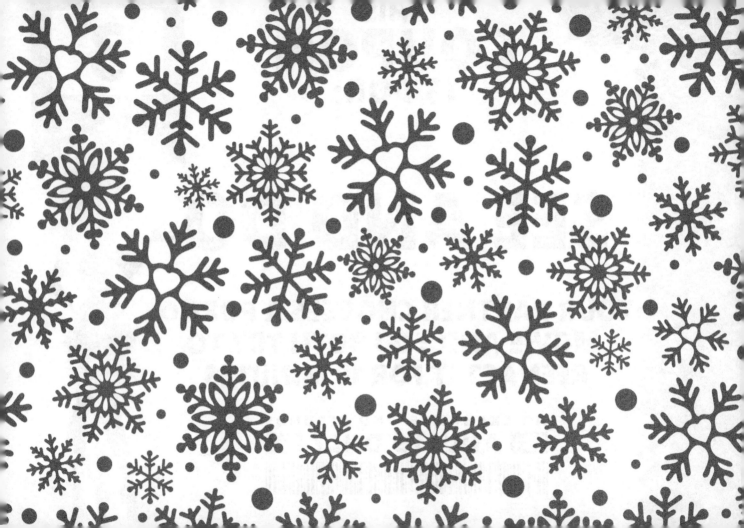

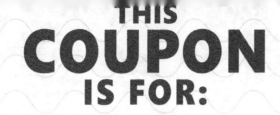

THIS
COUPON
IS FOR:

4

WILD
FANTASY

I WILL FULFILL ONE OF YOUR
INTIMATE FANTASIES

NO EXCHANGE - NO REFUNDS

18+ ADULTS ONLY 18+

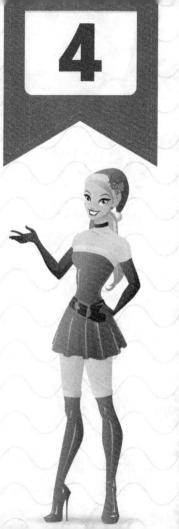

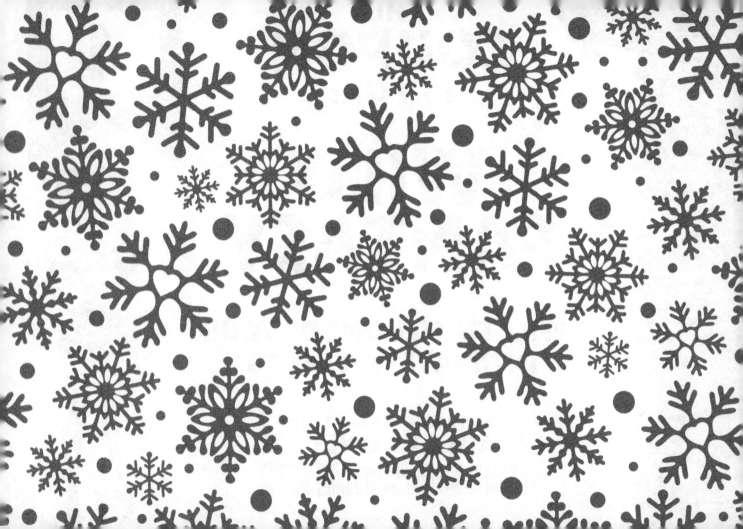

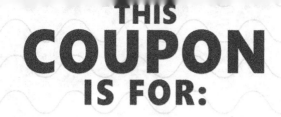

THIS
COUPON
IS FOR:

5

SUNDAY FUNDAY

AFTERNOON SEX EVERY SUNDAY FOR A MONTH

NO EXCHANGE - NO REFUNDS
18+ ADULTS ONLY 18+

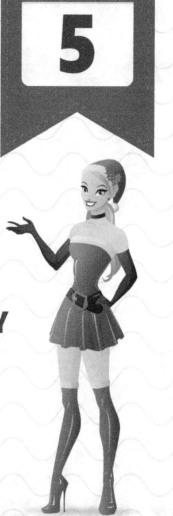

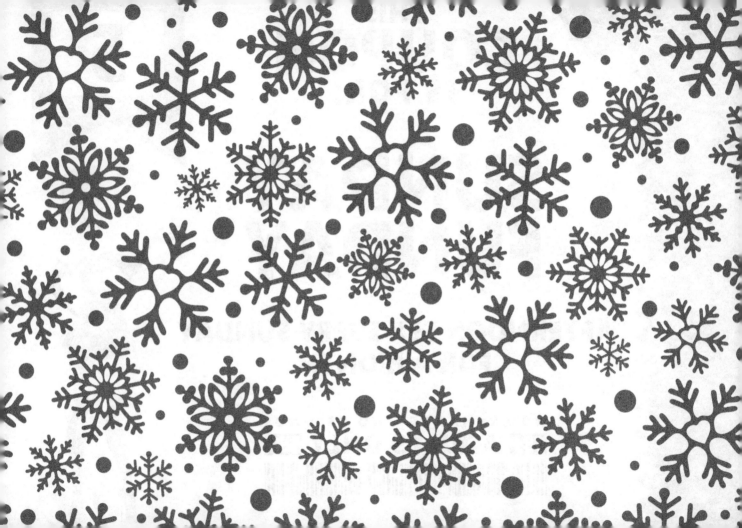

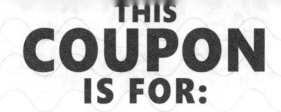

THIS COUPON IS FOR:

6

SENSUAL FOREPLAY

KEEP IT SLOW, TAKE IT EASY

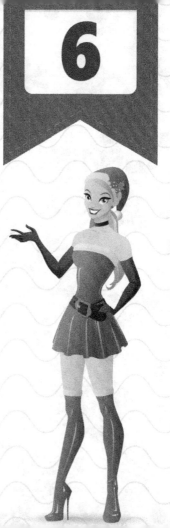

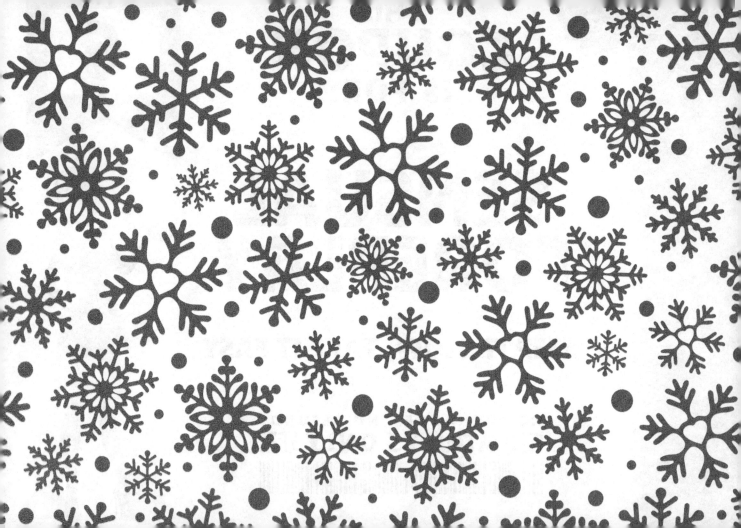

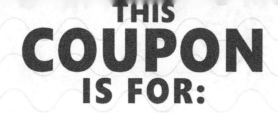

THIS
COUPON
IS FOR:

SENSUAL MASSAGE

NO CLOTHING REQUIRED

NO EXCHANGE - NO REFUNDS
18+ ADULTS ONLY 18+

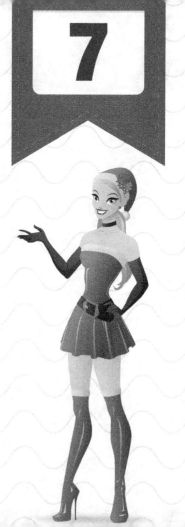

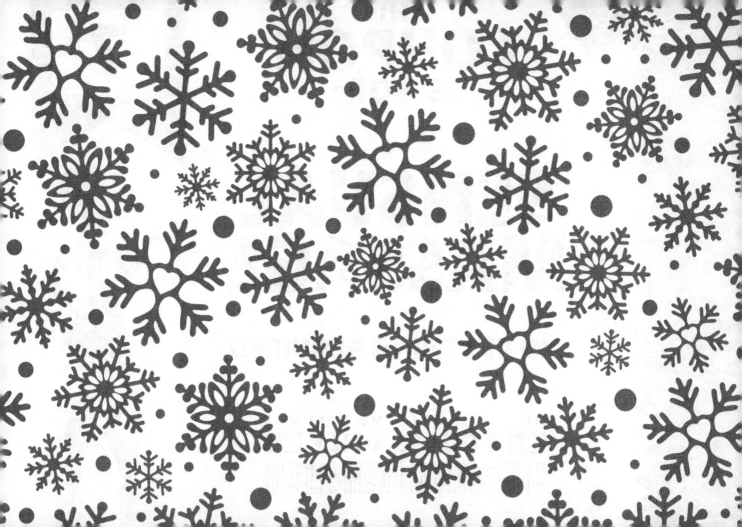

THIS COUPON IS FOR:

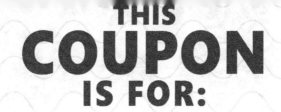

8

STEAMY SHOW FOR 2

WITH LOTS OF TOUCHING

NO EXCHANGE - NO REFUNDS
18+ ADULTS ONLY 18+

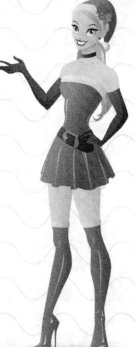

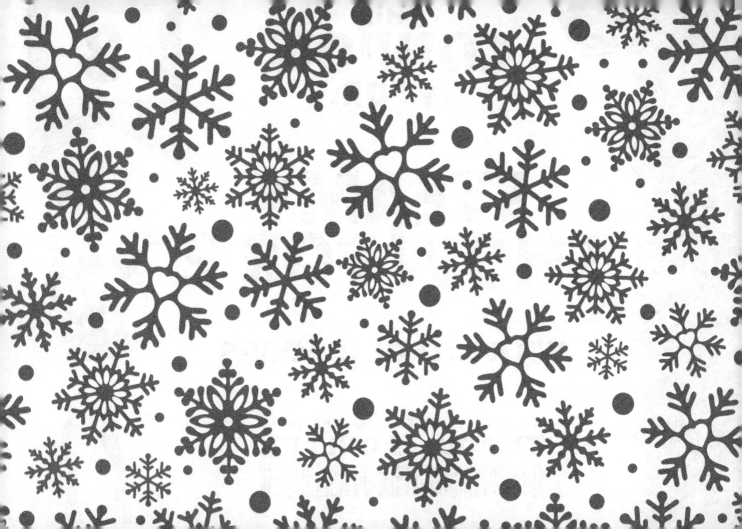

THIS
COUPON
IS FOR:

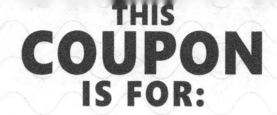

SEXY
PHOTO

SEND 1 SEXY PHOTO OF YOU
WITHIN THE NEXT 7 DAYS

NO EXCHANGE - NO REFUNDS
18+ ADULTS ONLY 18+

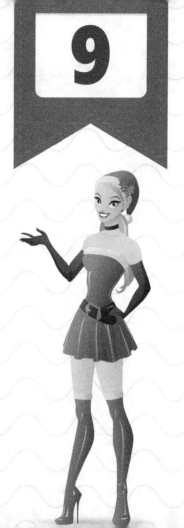

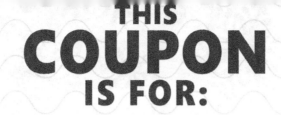

THIS
COUPON
IS FOR:

QUICKIE

LET'S GET IT ON!

NO EXCHANGE - NO REFUNDS
18+ ADULTS ONLY 18+

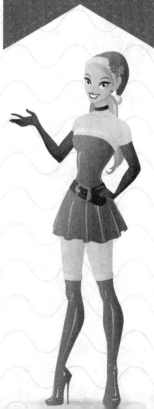

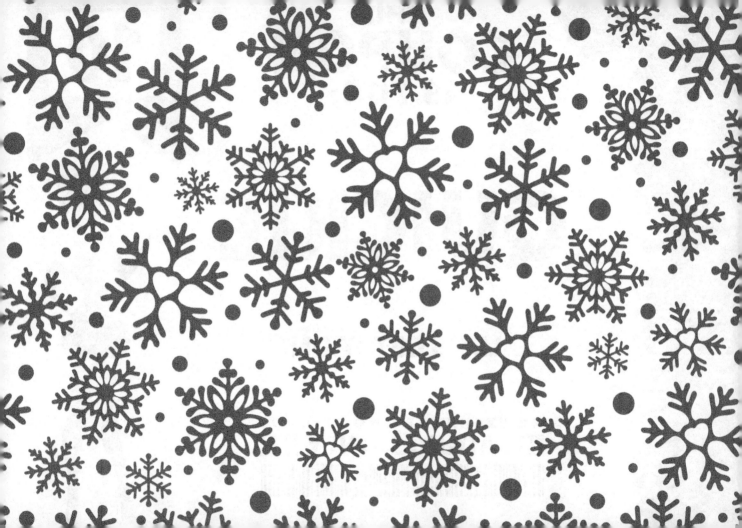

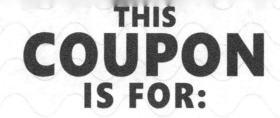

THIS
COUPON
IS FOR:

11

GOOD FOR
ANYTHING

VALID FOR ONE REQUEST

NO EXCHANGE - NO REFUNDS
18+ ADULTS ONLY 18+

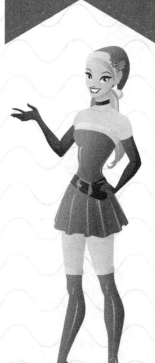

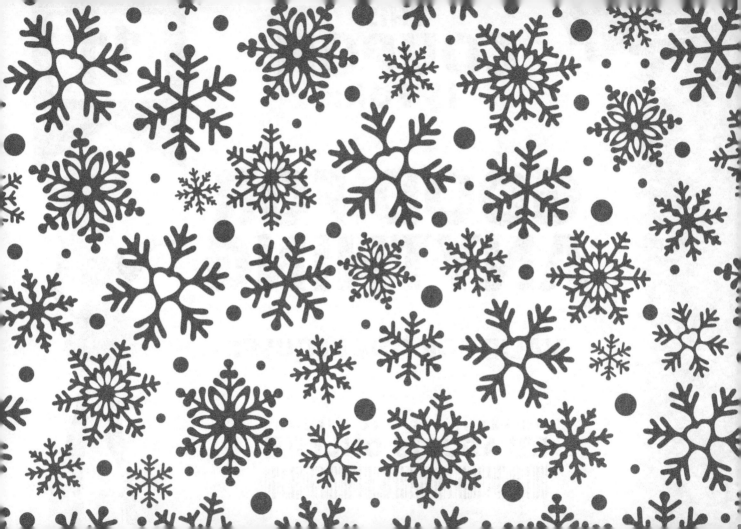

THIS COUPON IS FOR:

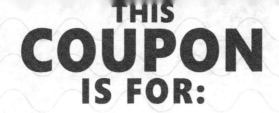

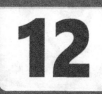

12

WAKE-UP SEX

WAKE HIM UP WITH ORAL PLEASURE

NO EXCHANGE - NO REFUNDS

18+ ADULTS ONLY 18+

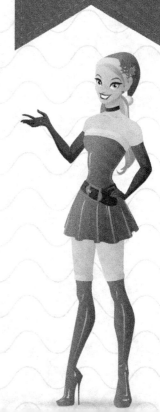

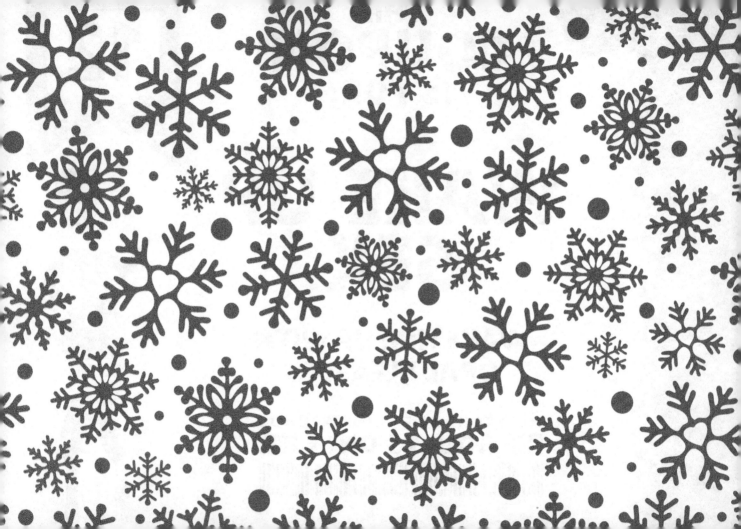

THIS COUPON IS FOR:

13

FIRST DATE RE-DO

LET'S RELIEVE OUR FIRST DATE

NO EXCHANGE - NO REFUNDS

18+ ADULTS ONLY 18+

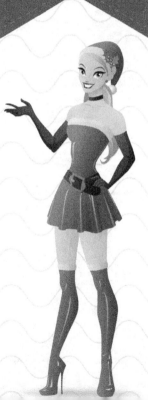

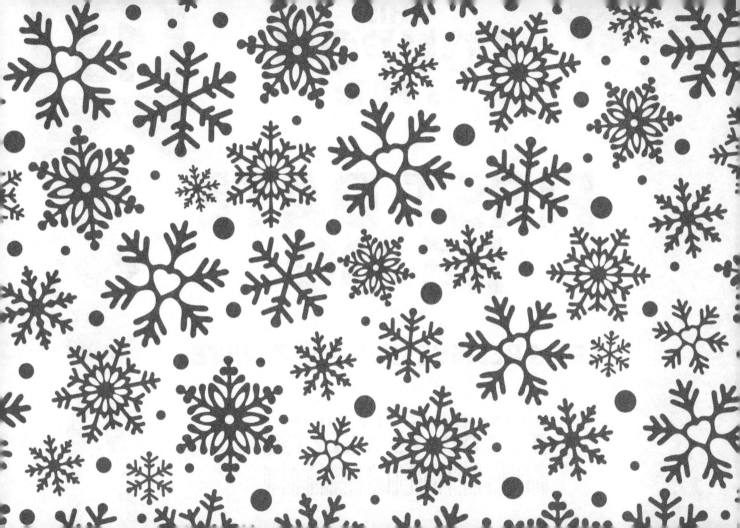

THIS COUPON IS FOR:

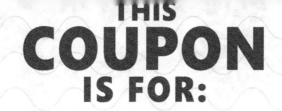

LAP DANCE

CLOTHING OPTIONAL

NO EXCHANGE - NO REFUNDS
18+ ADULTS ONLY 18+

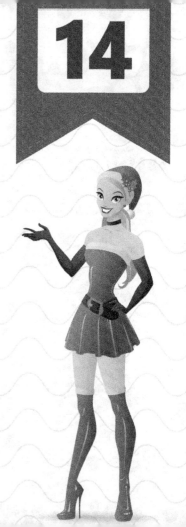

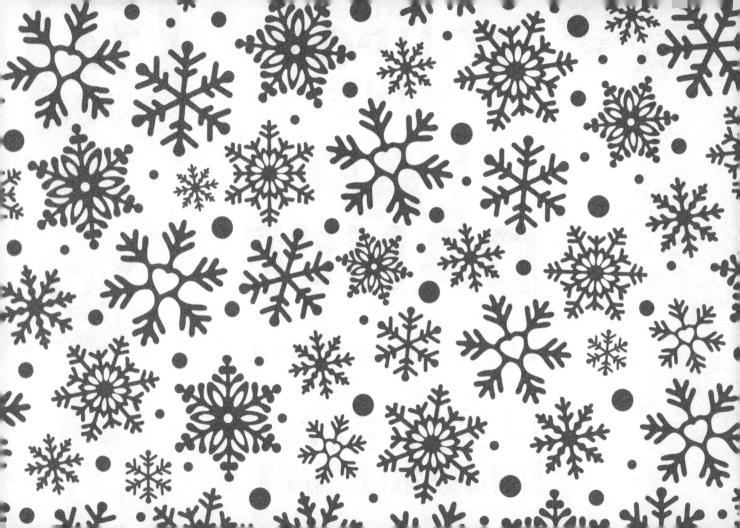

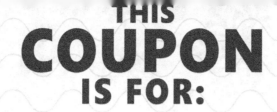

THIS
COUPON
IS FOR:

15

BREAKFAST
IN BED

COOK ME BREAKFAST
AND THEN JOIN ME

NO EXCHANGE - NO REFUNDS
18+ ADULTS ONLY 18+

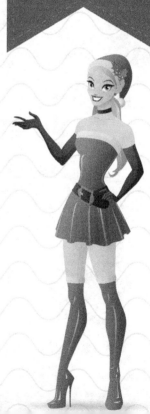

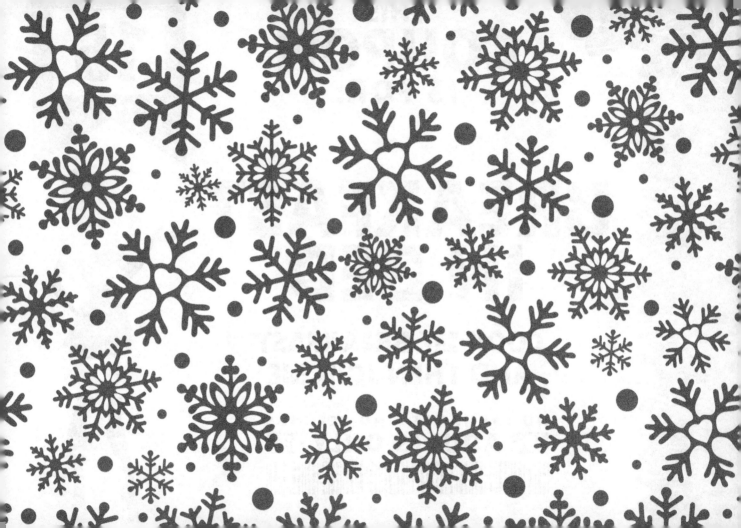

COUPON
IS FOR:

16

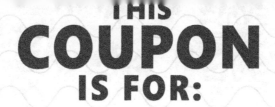

NIGHT OF
ROLE PLAY

SHOULD I BE A NURSE OR
A SEXY SECRETARY?

NO EXCHANGE - NO REFUNDS

18+ ADULTS ONLY 18+

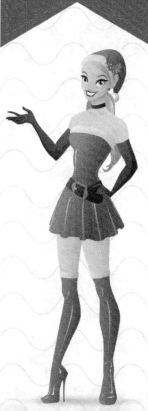

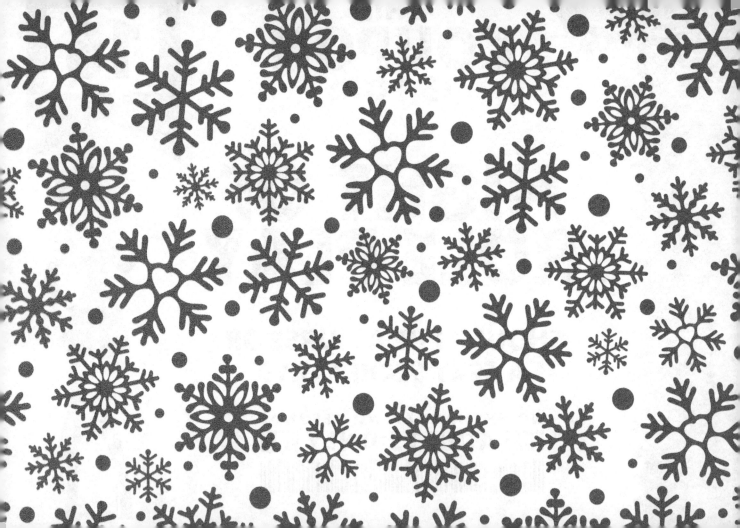

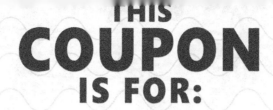

THIS
COUPON
IS FOR:

NAKED
MOVIE
NIGHT

BUT YOU CAN'T WATCH
WITHOUT TOUCHING

NO EXCHANGE - NO REFUNDS
18+ ADULTS ONLY 18+

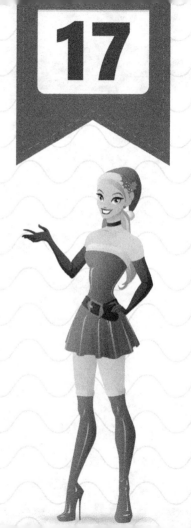

17

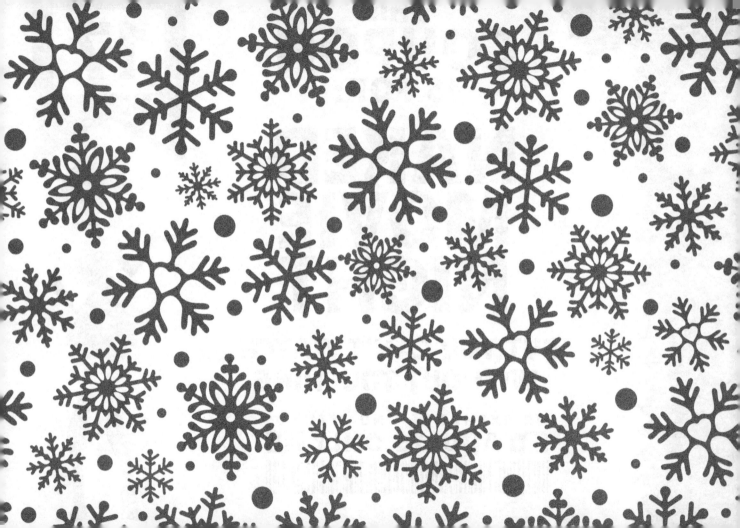

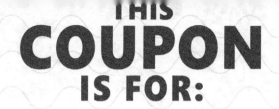

THIS COUPON IS FOR:

STRIP TEASE

**YOU PICK THE MUSIC
I PICK THE OUTFIT**

18

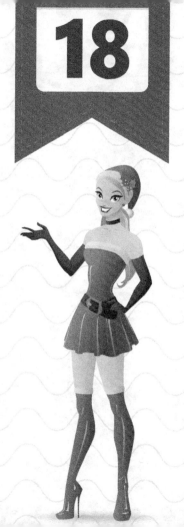

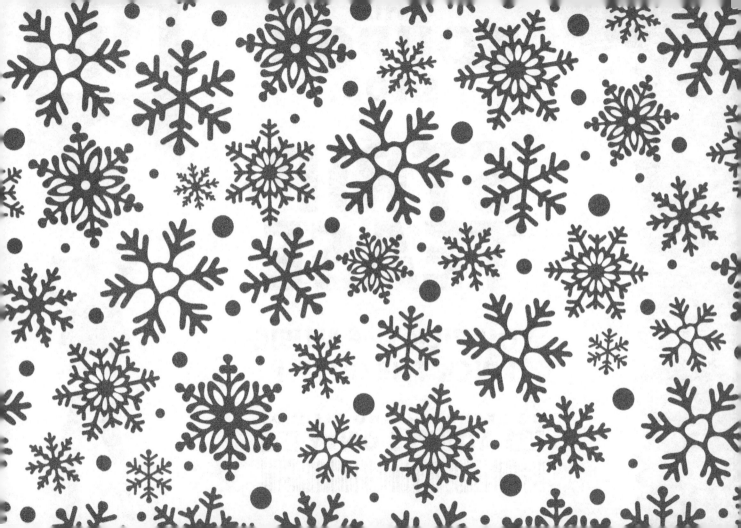

THIS
COUPON
IS FOR:

NEW POSITION

TIME TO TEST SOMETHING NEW

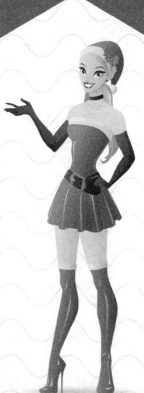

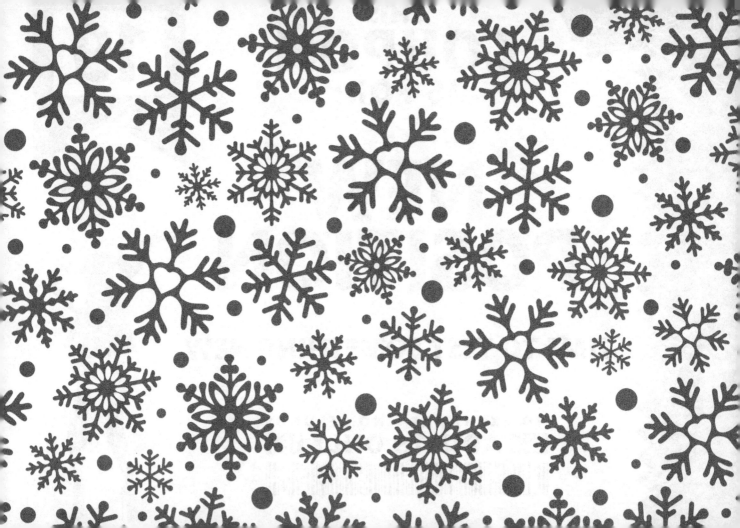

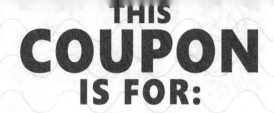

THIS COUPON IS FOR:

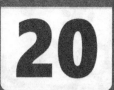

GOOSE-BUMPS

KISS AND LICK YOUR PARTNER'S BACK FROM BOTTON TO NECK. MAKE IT EXTRA EROTIC

NO EXCHANGE - NO REFUNDS

18+ ADULTS ONLY 18+

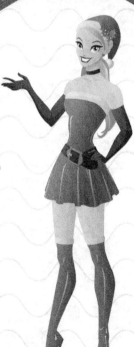

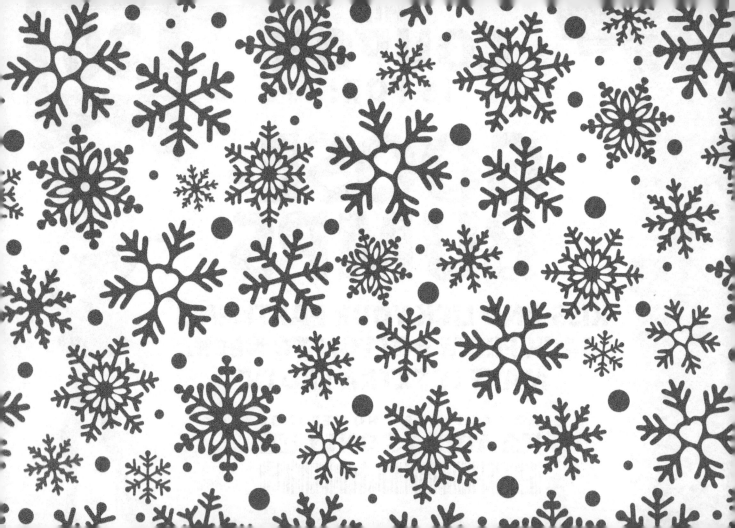

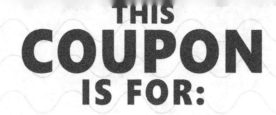

THIS COUPON IS FOR:

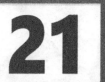

21

69

THIS ONE BENEFITS EVERYONE

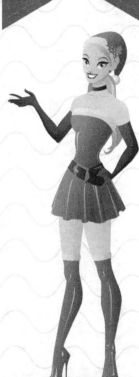

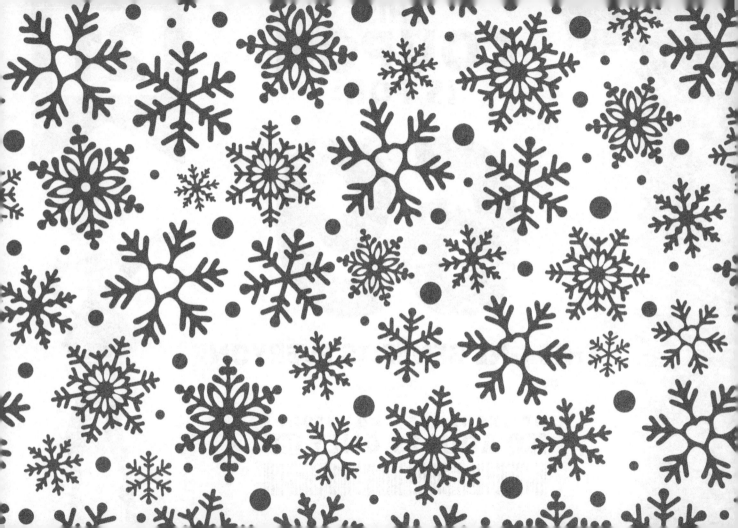

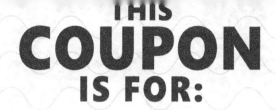

THIS COUPON IS FOR:

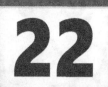

PLAY THE BOMB

SET A TIMER FOR 20 MINUTES, PLAY, KISS, AND DO WHATEVER YOU WANT, BUT NO PENETRATION IS ALLOWED UNTIL THE TIMER IS UP

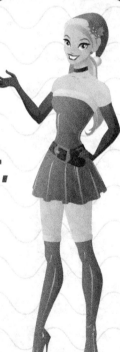

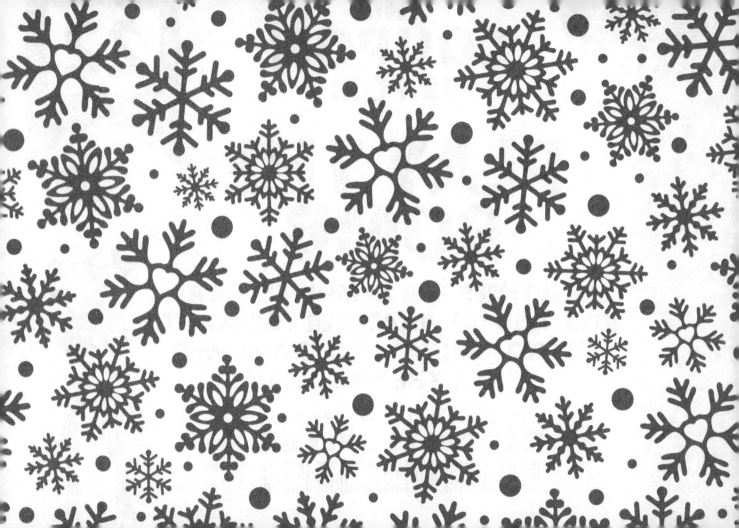

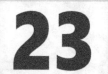

THIS
COUPON
IS FOR:

23

ANYTHING
YOU DESIRE

NO LIMITS!

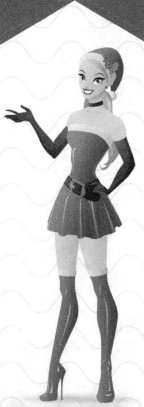

NO EXCHANGE - NO REFUNDS
18+ ADULTS ONLY 18+

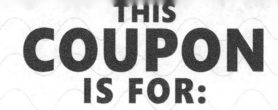

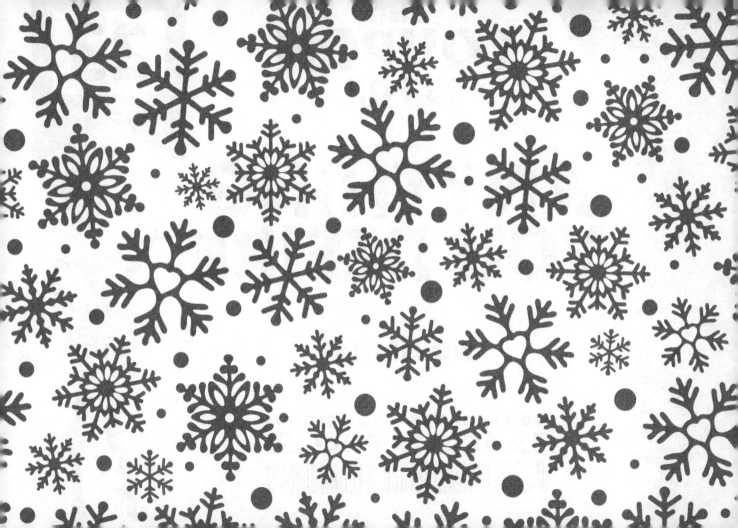

THIS COUPON IS FOR:

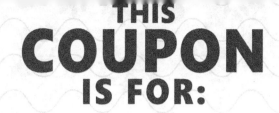

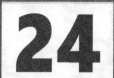

24

ONE ALL-NIGHTER

LET'S STAY UP AND STAY BUSY

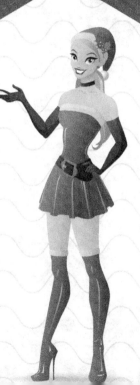

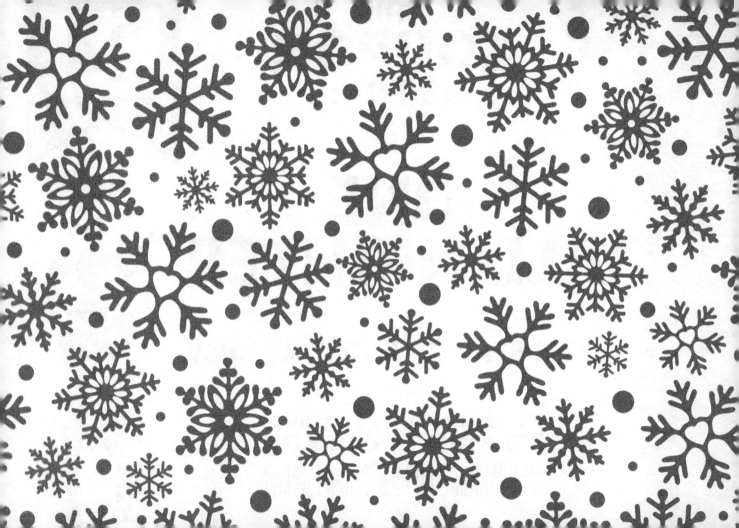

THIS
COUPON
IS FOR:

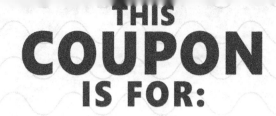

....

....

NO EXCHANGE - NO REFUNDS
18+ ADULTS ONLY 18+

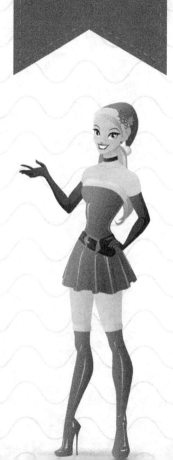

THIS
COUPON
IS FOR:

....

....

NO EXCHANGE - NO REFUNDS
18+ ADULTS ONLY 18+

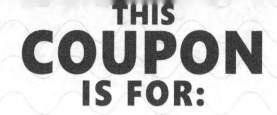

THIS
COUPON
IS FOR:

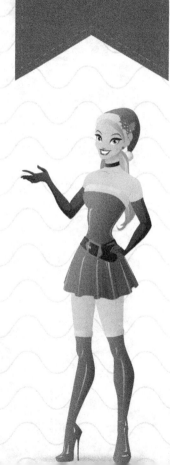

....

....

NO EXCHANGE - NO REFUNDS
18+ ADULTS ONLY 18+

|||||||||||||||||||||||||||||||||||||||||||

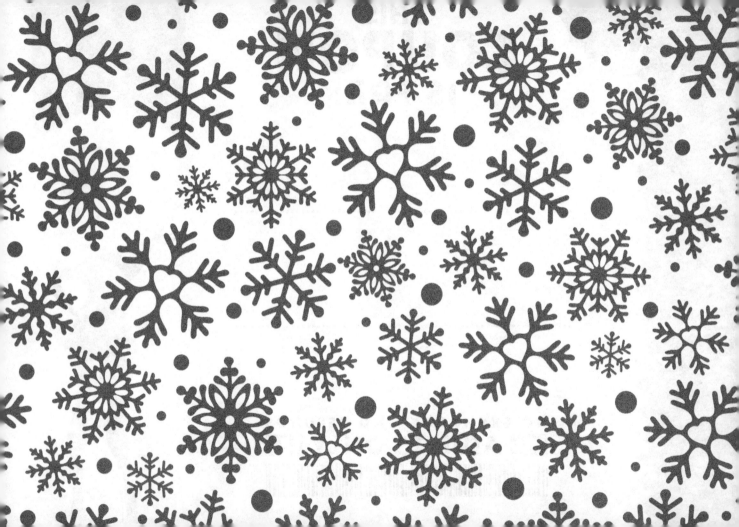

THIS
COUPON
IS FOR:

···

···

NO EXCHANGE - NO REFUNDS
18+ ADULTS ONLY 18+

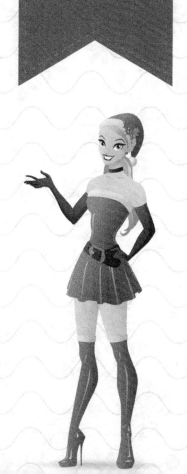

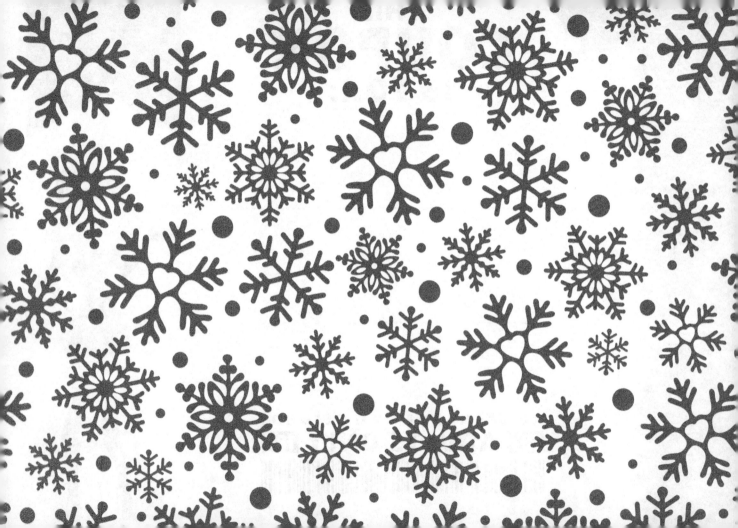

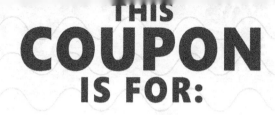

THIS
COUPON
IS FOR:

....

....

NO EXCHANGE - NO REFUNDS
18+ ADULTS ONLY 18+

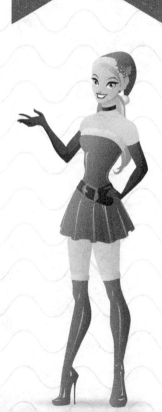

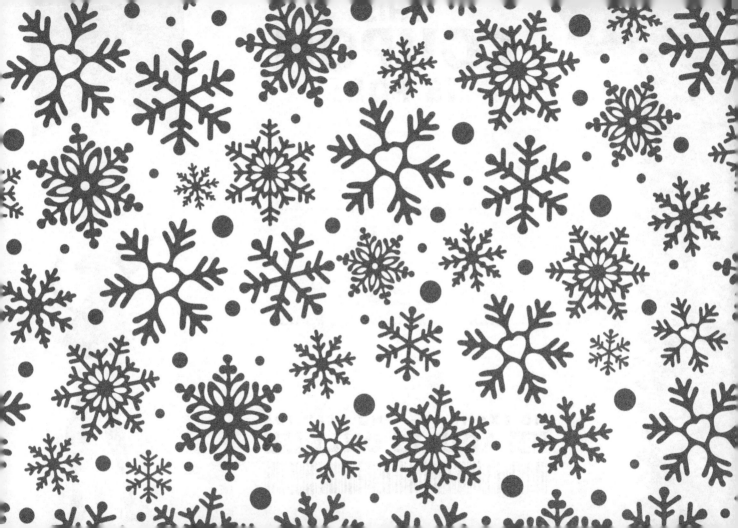

THIS
COUPON
IS FOR:

....

....

NO EXCHANGE - NO REFUNDS
18+ ADULTS ONLY 18+

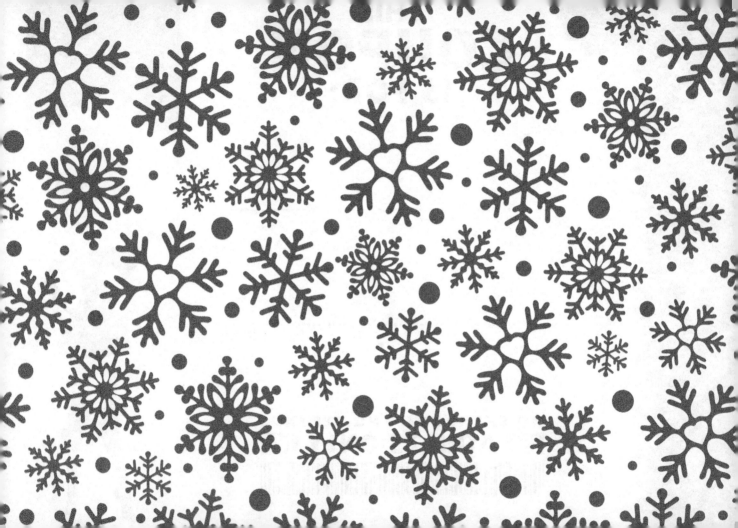

THIS
COUPON
IS FOR:

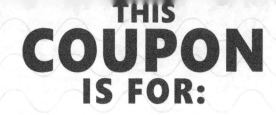

....

....

NO EXCHANGE - NO REFUNDS
18+ ADULTS ONLY 18+

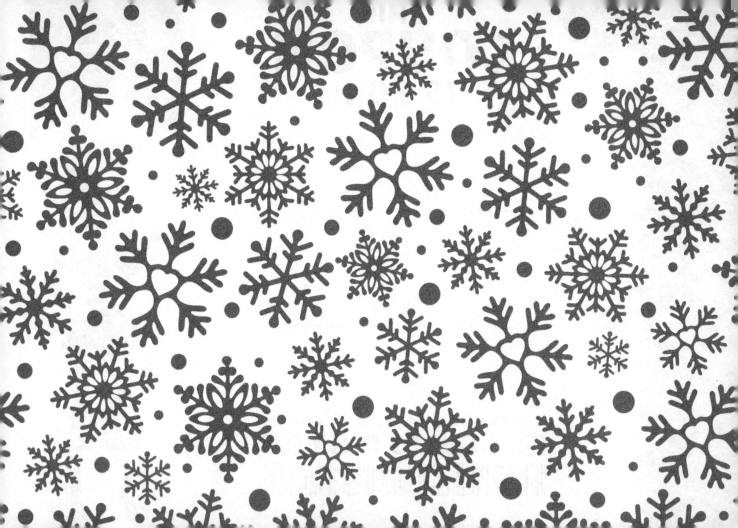

Made in the USA
Monee, IL
28 September 2023